MUSCULOSKELETAL ULTRASOUND:

THE ESSENTIALS

This text is dedicated to the memory of
my beloved mother Rhoswen Gibbon
who sadly died before its completion
from a long illness bravely borne.
You were greatly loved and are sorely missed.

MUSCULOSKELETAL ULTRASOUND:

THE ESSENTIALS

Dr WW Gibbon MB, BS, FRCS(Ed), FRCR

Consultant Skeletal Radiologist, The General Infirmary at Leeds

Hon. Clinical Senior Lecturer, University of Leeds

Director, The White Rose Institute of Sports Medicine, Leeds.

ᒐG\M\Mᒑ

© 1996
Greenwich Medical Media
507 The Linen Hall
162-168 Regent Street
London
W1R 5TB

ISBN 1 900 15105 7

First Published 1996

A catalogue record for this book is available from the British Library

Distributed worldwide by
Oxford University Press

Designed and Produced by
Derek Virtue, DataNet

Printed in Great Britain by
Derry Print Limited

CONTENTS

INTRODUCTION

Musculoskeletal ultrasound is an extremely useful and versatile technique for examining superficial soft-tissue pathology. Ultrasound has the advantages of being readily available and inexpensive, at the same time providing highly detailed information regarding superficial skeletal structures. The current concise text aims to provide, in pictorial form, the sonographic appearances of normal musculoskeletal structures as well as the more commonly encountered abnormalities. It is intended as a basic introduction into the exciting and, in many quarters underutilised, field of adult skeletal ultrasound.

Although skeletal ultrasound has been performed since the early 1970's its expansion was limited until recently due to the constraints of an ultrasound system's spatial resolution. The new generation of real-time ultrasound units coupled with great advances in transducer technology now allow exceptional superficial skeletal soft-tissue resolution which is slowly revolutionising our understanding of musculoskeletal pathology. Ultrasound in the future will increasingly provide knowledge not only as to the cause of a patient's symptoms but also the "cause of the cause", i.e. the underlying biomechanical problem.

It is often stated that skeletal ultrasound is operator-dependent with a steep and prolonged learning curve, which indeed is true, but not particularly more so than many other branches of imaging. Proficiency relates to good scanning technique and a detailed understanding of skeletal anatomy and pathology. It is always easier to see abnormalities when you know what structures you are looking at and what pathology you are looking for! However, it is becoming increasingly obvious to the author that you also require a good combination of ultrasound unit and high-resolution transducer in order to demonstrate those abnormalities. Skeletal ultrasound is thus equipment-dependent as much as operator-dependent. Indeed the more inexperienced an operator, the better an ultrasound system that is required for safe practice. The greatest danger of ultrasound is not its production of ionising radiation or thermal energy but in its providing an inaccurate diagnosis due to technical or operator limitations. At the present time inexpensive ultrasound systems probably do not have sufficient resolution for safe and accurate skeletal ultrasound - but this may change in the future.

A high-resolution linear array transducer is essential, preferably with a variable frequency of 10-5 MHz in order to provide good near-field resolution as well as tissue penetration for deeper structures. A 5 MHz transducer is however useful when examining deeper structure such as the adult hip (vide infra). The images in the current text were achieved using **ATL HDI 3000** or **Ultramark 9** units (**Advanced Technology Laboratories, Bothell, WA**) coupled in most cases with a 10-5 MHz 26mm or 38mm footprint linear-array transducer. A stand-off has not been used as these are not felt to be necessary when using these systems although liberal amounts of coupling gel may be required for demonstrating very superficial/subcutaneous structures.

A split-screen facility is extremely useful, especially for the inexperienced sonologist. Such a facility allows direct comparison with the contralateral limb which may help to avoid false-positive diagnoses, assuming that the opposite side is also normal and can act as an internal control (which is often not the case with overuse phenomena). Similarly it allows more accurate assessment of quantitative changes if strictly comparable images are achieved (such images being more readily compared if it is possible to include a bone surface in the image for localisation).

The text concentrates on adult conditions only. Childhood diseases e.g. hip dysplasias are beyond the scope of this current work.

TISSUE CHARACTERISTICS

The echogenicity of tissues varies with transducer frequency. At 10-5 MHz the tissues appear sonographically as below. The overall appearance may also reflect the echogenicity of adjacent tissues i.e. a structure may appear of low echogenicity (hypoechoic) when surrounded by bright (echogenic) tissues but relatively echogenic when surrounded by hypoechoic tissues.

Tendon: Tightly packed parallel longitudinally arranged collagen bundles result in a brightly echogenic structure with a fine internal fibrillar pattern.

Ligament: Sonographically, ligaments are similar to tendons except if more than one layer is present, e.g. medial ligament complex of knee, the fibrillar patterns of these layers may run in different directions.

Muscle: Hypoechoic muscle bundles are seen interspersed by the echogenic interfaces of epi- and para-mysium, with muscle compartments separated by echogenic connective tissue septae and investing fascia.

Fibrocartilage: Densely packed fibres result in a relatively homogenous structure although occasionally a subtle fibrillar pattern may be identified along the axis of the annularly arranged fibres.

Hyaline cartilage: Articular cartilage effectively contains no internal echoes in young adults (i.e. it is anechoic) but its echogenicity slowly increases with age especially if there is chondrocalcinosis.

Nerve: Similar to tendons but with much longer echogenic interfaces without interdigitations.

Adipose: The echogenicity of fat depends on the size of adipocytes. Fat itself does not usually contain interfaces therefore it is hypoechoic. Surrounding connective tissue, however, is echogenic. Therefore if adipocytes are small the overall appearance is of an echogenic structure whereas if they are large the tissue is hypoechoic.

Bone: The surface is usually brightly echogenic with profound posterior acoustic shadowing (unless bone is exceptionally thin e.g. squamous temporal bone in children).

In all cases a tissue's echogenicity varies with incident beam obliquity.

1: LS Sagittal Midline Anterior Knee

Split screen with the left-hand image demonstrating a normally echogenic patella tendon which in the right-hand image appears hypoechoic due to simply angling the transducer cephalad approximately 20 degrees to the tendon surface (arrowheads).

Diagnosis:

Normal tendon demonstrating "anisotropy" i.e. oblique beam artifact.

Key point:

Meticulous examination technique is essential to avoid errors. As will be explained most normal structures e.g. tendons, fibrocartilage and ligaments are echogenic or they are low echo structures interspersed with echogenic bands, e.g. skeletal muscle. Pathology, however, is usually hypoechoic due to oedema separating normal tissue interfaces and disruption of interfaces resulting in scatter. Unfortunately beam obliquity will result in artifactual decreased echogenicity (anisotropy) hence the need to maintain the beam perpendicular to the structure being examined at all times. This however does not mean being perpendicular to the skin surface as this may not be parallel to the structure in question. Similarly if a tendon is not examined under tension the central portion may be echogenic while the tendon at the periphery of the screen is artifactually hypoechoic (this being the same problem if a curved – rather than linear – array transducer is used to examine a linear structure).

2: LS Posterior Heel

Examination of the retro-calcaneal bursa region (arrowheads) both with and without compression demonstrating how the presence of small amounts of fluid within bursae, tendon sheaths etc may be missed if excessive transducer pressure is applied.

Key point:

When examining bursal regions care must be taken not to produce so much pressure on the bursa that its easily deformable walls become effaced and thus more difficult to identify. Such a compression phenomenon may be useful however when attempting to distinguish between complex fluid which is ballottable and synovial thickening which is relatively non-compressible.

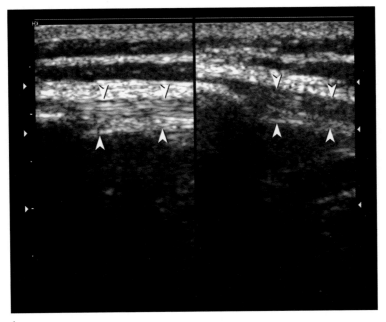

1

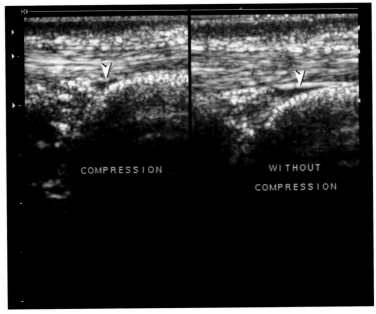

2

3: LS Posterior Heel

A thin layer of fluid is present within a non-distended superficial pre-calcaneal bursa (arrow-heads). The absence of surrounding low-echogenicity (i.e. oedema) makes active inflammation unlikely. Also the smooth convexity and bright echogenicity of the distal Achilles tendon show this structure also to be normal.

> **Key point:**
>
> The utilisation of a thick layer of contact medium and gentle transducer pressure allows clearer visualisation of near-field structures and also maintains good transducer contact when angulation is required.

4: LS Posterior Heel

A small amount of fluid in the retro-calcaneal bursa (curved arrow) may not be abnormal in isolation but can provide a pointer as to an underlying biomechanical dysfunction when associated with other "normal" appearances such as a posterior calcaneal spur (S). A notch (arrows) on the posterior calcaneal surface reflects the proximal Achilles calcaneal insertion, the tendon normally demonstrating a smooth convexity from this point down to its distal limit of attachment. A posterior calcaneal spur would appear to reflect the body's attempt at shortening the tendon's excursion, thus presumably reducing its vertical tension forces. The decreased echogenicity of the distal tendon insertion (arrowheads) is likely to be artifactual due in part to anisotropy as the collagen bundles change from a vertical to a more horizontal alignment as they approach their calcaneal insertion.

> **Key points:**
>
> 1) A larger footprint transducer may provide a better global overview of such regions (although there may be slight decrease in spatial resolution).
>
> 2) If, however, decreased echogenicity persists at tendon insertions it may reflect inflammation in region of Sharpey-Shaffer fibres, e.g. in sero-negative arthropathies.

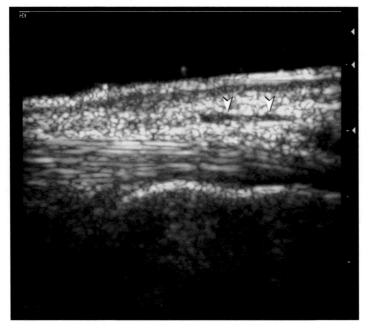

3

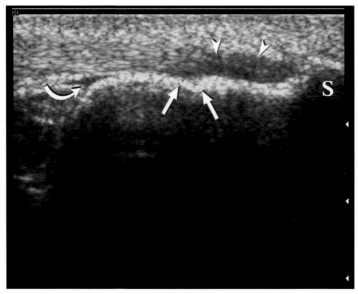

4

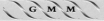

5: LS Posterior Heel

Normal calcaneus (C) without surface erosion and a retro-calcaneal bursa (arrows) which is distended with fluid and has a thickened wall demonstrating finger-like internal projections and surrounding oedema. The Achilles paratenon (arrowheads) is thickened, hypoechoic and ill-defined consistent with active inflammation. The distal Achilles tendon is also thickened and of decreased/heterogenous echogenicity consistent with a distal third tendonitis.

The acoustic shadowing at the proximal bursal margin could reflect crystal deposition but may be artifactual due to high acoustic impedance difference interface and scatter (similar changes are often seen at the ends of a ruptured tendon).

Diagnosis:

Retro-calcaneal bursitis with both distal Achilles tendonitis and paratendonitis without calcaneal erosion.

Key point:

When bursae enlarge they usually do so away from point of maximum pressure producing a tear-drop appearance with its neck at site of original compression.

6: TS Middle Third Achilles Tendons

The right Achilles tendon (R) is a normal oblique ellipse containing multiple echogenic dots reflecting end-on collagen bundles. The left Achilles tendon (L) is more rounded in cross-section with a thickened surrounding hypoechoic paratenon (arrowheads). The deep portion of the tendon in particular demonstrates a more heterogenous pattern.

Diagnosis:

Chronic Achilles tendonitis and paratendonitis.

Key point:

Achilles tendon thickening is almost inevitably more marked in its antero-posterior than its transverse diameter (similarly the patella tendon).

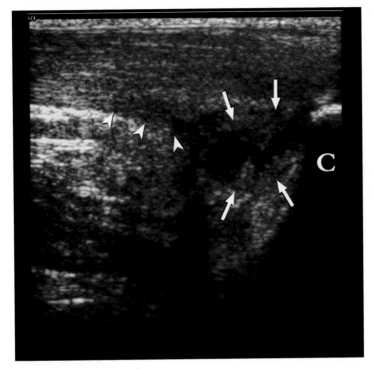

5

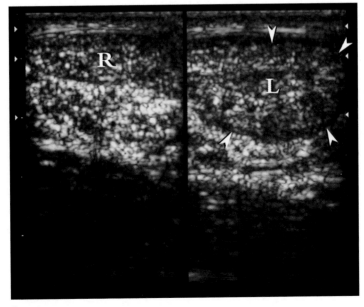

6

7a: TS Middle Third Achilles Tendon
7b: LS Middle Third Achilles Tendon

There is a focal area of decreased echogenicity superficial/medial aspect of mid–Achilles tendon (arrowheads, 7a) with a localised bulge to the superficial or subcutaneous border (arrowheads, 7b). The deep and lateral segments appear normal in both planes. There is no associated paratenon (nor bursal) abnormality.

Diagnosis:

Focal or nodular chronic Achilles tendonitis.

Key points:

1) Proximal/middle third Achilles tendon disease is usually secondary to an underlying biomechanical abnormality.

2) Although usually termed "tendonitis" the primary problem is degenerative with attempted repair, i.e. tendinosis rather than inflammation (whereas distal third Achilles tendonitis is usually inflammatory and therefore a true tendonitis).

3) The distribution of focal or nodular tendon disease will often suggest the nature of underlying biomechanical problem :-

   i) Medial segment - heel hyperpronation.

   ii) Superficial segment - footwear impingement or reduced ankle dorsiflexion.

   iii) Deep segment - significance unclear but again likely to reflect increased focal longitudinal stresses.

   iv) Distal tendon - deep surface impingement in full dorsiflexion by prominent posterior-superior calcaneal tubercle.

4) Similar but usually milder changes are often present on examination of the patient's contra-lateral Achilles tendon even when asymptomatic.

5) Patterns may be combinations of the above.

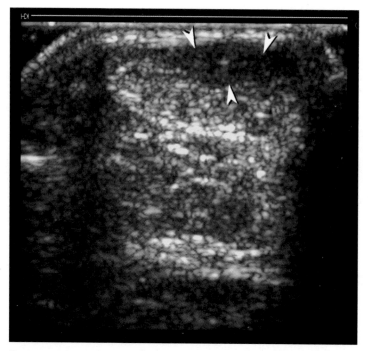

7a

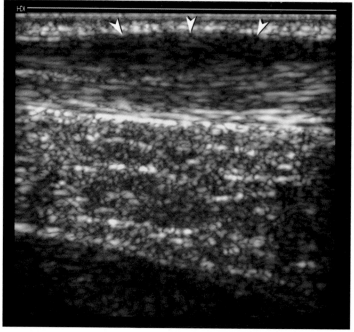

7b

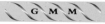

8a: TS Middle Third Achilles Tendon
8b: LS Middle Third Achilles Tendon

There is a focus of almost anechoic tissue (arrows) within a diffusely decreased/hetero-genous deep portion of tendon (arrowheads) and a normal superficial tendon. The contour of the deep surface is becoming irregular.

Diagnosis:

Severe tendon degeneration / intrasubstance tear.

Key points:

1) The focus of very low echogenicity is likely to reflect either a small area of mucoid degeneration or frank tear within the more diffuse area of degeneration.

2) When there is a localised surface irregularity or discontinuity it is likely that a true partial tear exists.

3) It is likely that severe tendinosis, intrasubstance tear, partial thickness tear and complete rupture are different points in the spectrum of the same disease process.

4) In patients with tendon rupture 90-95% of contra-lateral Achilles tendons also exhibit sonographic changes of tendon disease.

5) Early diagnosis of the specific biomechanical abnormality predisposing to Achilles tendon disease may allow correction of the abnormality by simple conservative measures before the stage of frank tear is reached.

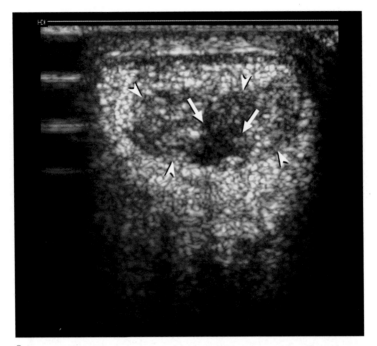

8a

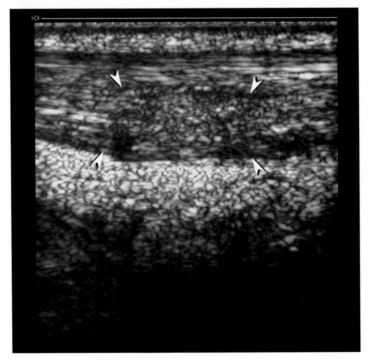

8b

9: LS Middle Third Achilles Tendon

There is a grossly abnormal Achilles tendon (A) which demonstrates generalised decreased echogenicity and rounded overlapping ends separated by an isthmus of echogenic fat (arrowheads). There is no peritendinous oedema or haemorrhage.

Diagnosis:

Ununited Achilles tendon rupture.

Key points:

1) The absence of surrounding oedema or haemorrhage combined with rounded and overlapping tendon ends suggests that the rupture is not recent.

2) The interposition of fat from Kager's triangle between tendon ends makes healing without surgical intervention unlikely.

3) If a normal plantaris tendon is present dynamic study may still demonstrate ankle plantar-flexion.

4) A plantaris tendon is present in approximately 90% of the general population, but in only 50-60% of patients with Achilles tendon rupture, suggesting a protective effect due to load redistribution.

5) The plantaris tendon lies medial and deep to the Achilles tendon (better seen in disease).

10: LS Medial Para-Sagittal Inferior Heels

A split-screen facility has been used to compare the normal left (L) and abnormal right (R) heels. The term "plantar fascia" is a misnomer and is more correctly termed the common tendinous aponeurosis of the superficial layer of intrinsic plantar muscles. The normal left plantar aponeurosis insertion (P) is echogenic similar to tendons elsewhere in the body. The right plantar aponeurosis is thickened and of heterogenous/decreased echogenicity (arrowheads). A sharp anterior cut-off to the inferior calcaneal tubercle is present on the right (arrow) when compared to the smoother left anterior border.

Diagnosis:

Plantar "fascitis" and inferior calcaneal spur formation.

Key points:

1) The plantar aponeurosis is normally thicker medially and has a maximum thickness of <4mm where it crosses the inferior/anterior calcaneal border.

2) A thickness of >4.5mm or a thickness difference of >1mm between sides is abnormal.

3) A subcalcaneal spur lies anterior and deep to the plantar aponeurosis origin, i.e. it is a buttressing not a traction phenomenon.

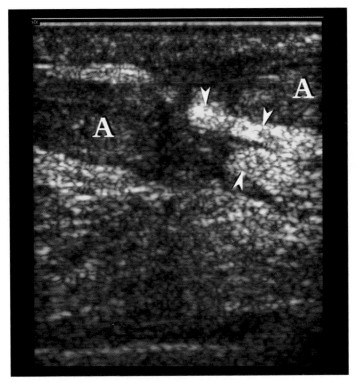

9

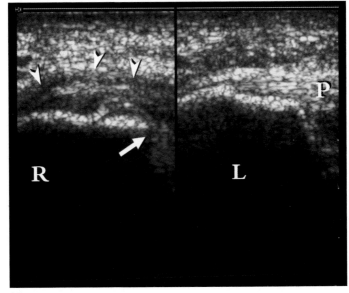

10

11a: TS Left Posterior Tibial Tendon

The tibialis posterior tendon is thickened with heterogenous/decreased echogenicity generally and a focal area of more marked low echogenicity (curved arrow). The tendon sheath is distended with fluid. These changes are at the posterior border of medial malleolus (M). No effusion is present in the space between the medial malleolus and talus (T).

Diagnosis:

Posterior tibial tenosynovitis and tendonitis with possible longitudinal tear.

11b: TS Oblique Anterior Medial (Deltoid) Ankle Ligament

The superficial portion of the deltoid ligament is seen as a markedly hypoechogenic band lying superficial to the tip of medial malleolus (M) and antero–medial border of talus (T). The distal section of the deep ligament is of more normal echogenicity (arrowheads) and is separated from the talus by a thin hypoechoic line of synovium/capsule again without evidence of ankle joint effusion.

Diagnosis:

Diffuse tear of the superficial and proximal tear of the deep component of medial ligament complex.

Key points:

1) There is a tear of the static medial ankle stabiliser, i.e. medial ankle ligament complex.

2) Secondary degenerative changes are present in one of the dynamic medial ankle stabilisers, i.e. posterior tibial tendon, as it attempts to compensate for the medial ankle instability due to extensive medial ligament complex injury.

3) Posterior tibial (and peroneal) tendon tears often occur at the level of the malleoli and are typically oblique longitudinal tears at this level reflecting the underlying abnormal shear forces.

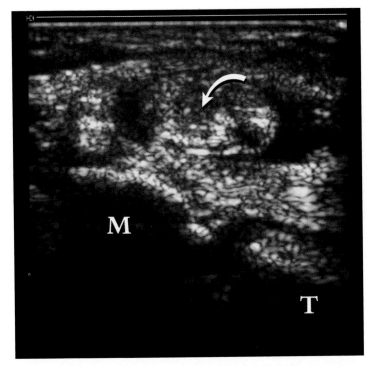

11a

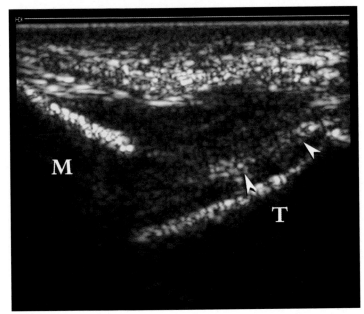

11b

12: LS Coronal Medial Ankle

The ossified medial aspects of the distal tibial metaphysis (M) and talus (T) are clearly identifiable either side of the ossified (E) and non-ossified cartilage of the medial malleolus epiphysis. A small triangle of fluid lies in the angle between the deep surface of the medial malleolus, medial border of talus and the deep portion of the medial deltoid ligament (D). A normal fleck of calcification (arrow) is present within the otherwise non-ossified structural cartilage eccentric to the main ossific nucleus. A reverberation echo (curved arrow) is present between the tibial metaphysis and epiphysis representing the area of the distal tibial physeal plate.

Diagnosis:

Normal skeletally immature ankle (boy aged 10 years).

Key point:

Ultrasound is an excellent, if underutilised method of assessing potential injury to non-ossified structural cartilage and the other structures around the "growing end" of bone/joints.

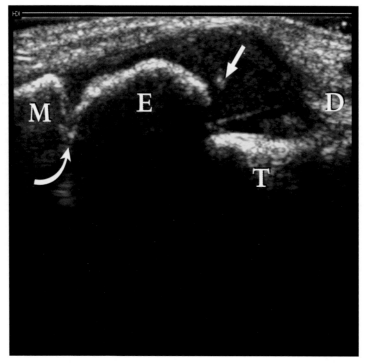

12

13a: Sagittal LS and Oblique TS Right Hip (7-4 MHz)
13b: Oblique TS Right Hip (10-5 MHz)

The anterior joint capsule is echogenic particularly at its superficial interface and separated from the femoral head (F) by a thin hypoechoic layer of hyaline articular cartilage. This cartilage layer is much more clearly identified at higher frequency (Fig 13b) but unfortunately in most adults the hip joint is too deep to use such a high frequency transducer.

The echogenic acetabular labrum (arrow) is clearly identified in the interspace between the femoral head and the bony acetabulum (A).

Diagnosis:

Normal study.

Key points:

Examination of hips is preferably performed with the patient's medial malleoli regions in contact, this symmetrical position allowing ready comparison of contra-lateral hips. A discrepancy of 1mm or more in the capsular-femoral distance should be considered to be significant.

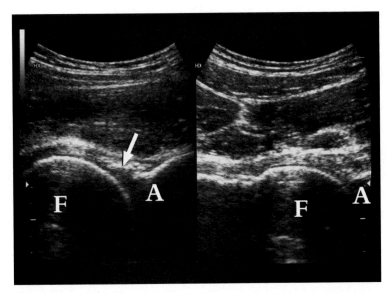

13a

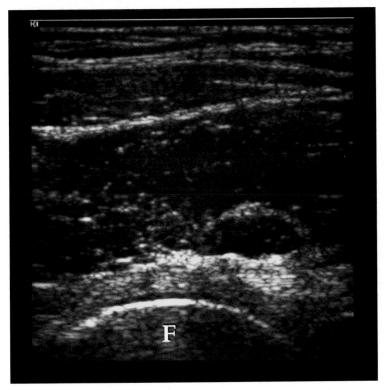

13b

14: LS Coronal Medial Knee

The superficial interface of the proximal attachment medial collateral ligament is more convex than normal (arrowheads) with loss of the normal echogenic fibrillar pattern seen more distally (M). The area of the combined deep and superficial medial collateral ligaments to the medial femoral condyle is thus thickened and of fusiform decreased/ heterogenous echogenicity.

Diagnosis:

Sprain of the femoral origin medial collateral ligament of knee.

Key point:

Although tears may occur at any point along its length, it is the author's experience that the femoral attachment is the commonest site for isolated tears.

15: LS Coronal Medial Knee

There is decreased echogenicity and thickening of the superficial layer of the proximal medial collateral ligament (arrowheads) with relatively normal deep layer (curved arrows). An area of acoustic shadowing is present extending through the ligament at its femoral attachment (C). This area of apparent calcification appears to be within the ligament rather than at its deep/femoral surface suggesting intra-ligamentous calcification and not ligament avulsion.

Diagnosis:

Pelligrini-Stieda lesion secondary to medial collateral ligament tear.

Key point:

There is no effusion in the medial femoral recess making intra-articular injury unlikely, however, ultrasound is unable to directly assess accurately and thus exclude possible associated cruciate ligament injury. Ultrasound can occasionally demonstrate associated peripheral detachments of the medial meniscus.

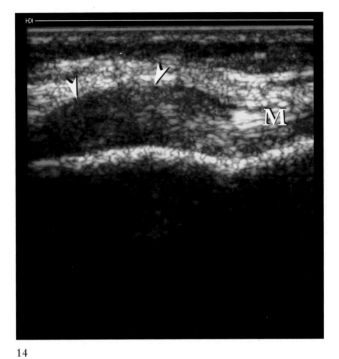

14

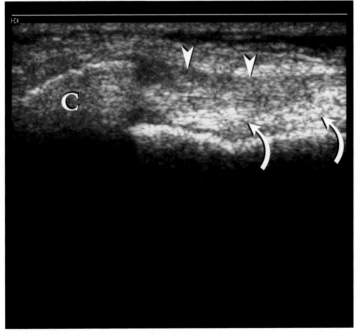

15

16: LS and TS wood foreign body in subcutaneous tissue of lateral knee

Split screen image showing on the left the two right interfaces of superficial and deep surface of a wood foreign body. There is very little in the way of acoustic shadowing but granulomatous reaction is present both at its proximal and distal end. This is best seen in the left-hand image with the foreign body in longitudinal section but in transverse section (right-hand image) the double interface and surrounding hypoechoic granulation tissue is again identified.

Diagnosis:

Wood foreign body.

Key points:

1) The lack of acoustic shadowing suggests a relatively low acoustic impedence material. There is no reverberation echo to suggest the foreign body to be either metal or glass.

2) Foreign bodies when recently penetrated through skin can be difficult to see due to artefact from air within the subcutaneous tissues producing reverberation echoes. Foreign bodies are better seen after they have been present for some time, particularly if they are producing (as in the above case) foreign body giant cell reaction or if the foreign body is producing a surrounding abscess collection of low echogenicity material.

17: LS Sagittal Midline Patella Tendon Origin

The proximal patella tendon (PT) has a broad patella origin with a slightly convex superficial surface. There is a longitudinal fissure at the tendon origin within an otherwise normal tendon (arrowheads).

Diagnosis:

Patella tendon shear injury.

Key points:

A similar presumed shearing injury is occasionally seen in the Achilles tendon, particularly in footballers.

1) Focal tendon changes localised to medial or lateral sides is unusual but if present suggests significant malalignment of the extensor mechanism.

2) Localised distal tendon changes may be seen in patella insertion tendonitis associated with pre-tibial bursitis or, in adolescents, Osgood–Schlatter disease.

3) Diffuse, generalised changes occur in more advanced disease and also in patella tendons following knee arthroplasty.

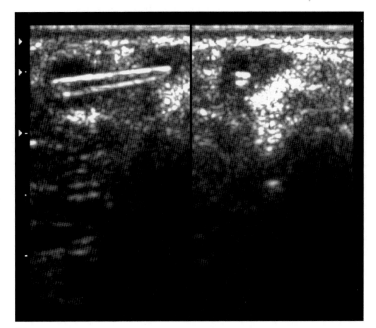

16

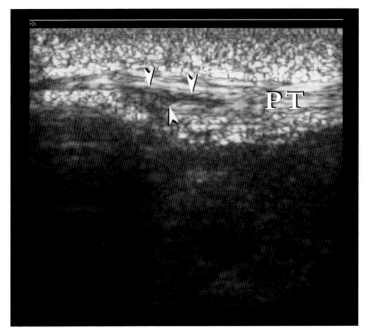

17

18: LS Sagittal Midline Patella Tendon Origin

A fissure is present in the surface of the inferior pole of patella (arrow). A very small calcific focus (curved arrow) is present within a decreased/heterogenous echogenicity deep surface of the patella tendon origin with a normal band of tendon more superficially.

Diagnosis:

1) Traction injury inferior pole of patella/Sinding-Larsen disease.

2) Patella tendonitis/Jumper's knee.

Key points:

1) In skeletal immaturity a hypoechoic area of non-ossified cartilage may be seen superficial to the ossified bone surface. These changes combined with thickening +/- irregularity of this non-ossified layer suggest Sinding-Larsen disease.

2) A focal area of tendonitis on the deep surface of the patella tendon, in the midline at the inferior pole of patella is typical of jumper's knee. In severe cases there may also be fluid demonstrated in a small adjacent bursa.

19: TS Mid Left Patella Tendon

The "echogenic dot" pattern seen in normal tendons on transverse section is seen medial half of patella tendon (P). The lateral half of the tendon is thickened and has lost this normal pattern (arrowheads). This latter region is of decreased/heterogenous echogenicity.

Diagnosis:

Focal lateral patella tendonitis.

Key point:

The above pattern is much less common than the "jumper's knee" changes of the midline patella tendon origin. The focal nature of the changes over the lateral half of the patella tendon implies increased forces in this region, possibly related to knee extensor mechanism malalignment. Occasionally similar isolated changes occur medially.

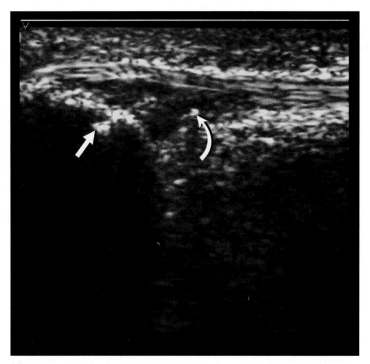

18

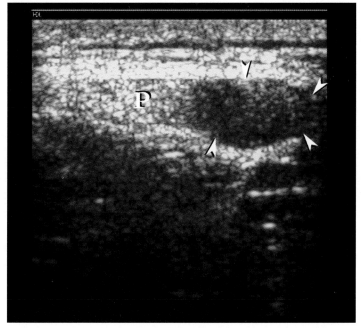

19

20: LS Coronal Medial Knee Joint

There is an area of echogenic reverberation echo ("comet-tail" artifact) deep to an echogenic interface consistent with changes seen at a soft-tissue/metal interface (M). Adjacent to this is an echogenic interface with posterior acoustic shadowing (P) this shadowing being incomplete there being a further interface below (curved arrow). The incomplete acoustic shadowing reflects the high-density polyethylene of the tibial component of a total knee replacement (TKR). The deeper interface seen through the plastic component also exhibits a faint reverberation echo and reflects the medial border of the metallic femoral component of the resurfacing TKR. These interfaces lie between the acoustic shadowing of the medial femoral condyle (F) and the prominence of the extruded bone cement (C) and medial tibial plateau (T).

Diagnosis:

Normal Total Knee Replacement.

Key point:

The fact that metalware produces susceptibility artifact around a joint replacement on MRI and streak artifact on CT, means ultrasound is finding increasing use in the assessment of soft-tissue abnormalities superficial to joint replacement, e.g. infective and wear-debris granulomata, abscesses and impingement problems, adventitial bursae, etc.

21: LS Coronal Medial Knee

Split-screen image demonstrates the advantage of dynamic or stress imaging. In the right-hand image scanning is being performed statically, i.e. at rest. The medial meniscus (M) appears small (which it often is medially in the true coronal plane) but otherwise normal. In the left-hand image a valgus strain has been applied while scanning the knee in order to open-up the medial joint space. The free edge of the meniscus is now much more clearly demonstrable.

Diagnosis:

The normal medial meniscus.

Key point:

Echoes are present deep within the medial knee compartment during stressing (arrows). These reflect reverberation echoes of gas bubbles within the synovial fluid and are akin to the vacuum phenomenon seen on stress radiography. These echoes can be seen to move with joint movement. Care should be taken not to misinterpret these echoes as being small loose bodies/debris.

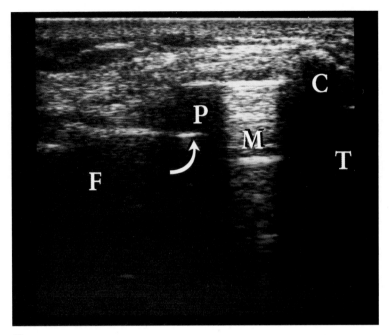

20

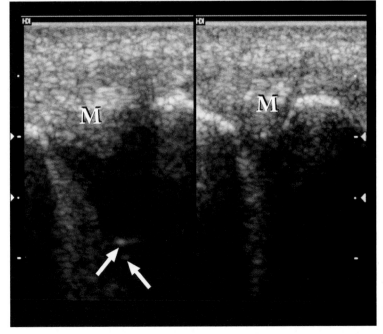

21

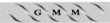

22a: LS Coronal Oblique Antero-Medial Knee

The medial meniscus (M) has an irregular, truncated free border (arrowheads). Echogenic material (arrows) is present within the triangular fluid space between the antero-medial aspect of medial femoral condyle (F) and medial tibial plateau (T).

22b: LS Coronal Oblique Antero-Medial Knee

   (10mm posterior to Fig 22a)

A horizontal fissure is present within the medial meniscus (curved arrow) and an osteophyte (O) is present at the periphery or the tibial plateau articular margin.

Diagnosis:

Two possibilities exist :-

1) There is a complex medial meniscal tear with horizontal cleavage tear and displaced "bucket-handle" tear components.

2) There has been a partial menisectomy for a horizontal cleavage tear of the medial meniscus.

In addition there are osteoarthritic changes and debris within the medial knee compartment.

Key points:

1) Ultrasound is able to clearly demonstrate the periphery of menisci anteriorly but may have difficulty demonstrating the posterior meniscal horns when a lower frequency transducer is required for depth of sound penetration in a large knee. Also due to the geometry of the knee articular surfaces it is usually difficult to demonstrate the entire meniscal free edge.

2) Regardless of these limitations ultrasound can demonstrate clearly meniscal cysts as well as associated horizontal cleavage tears and also peripheral meniscal detachments.

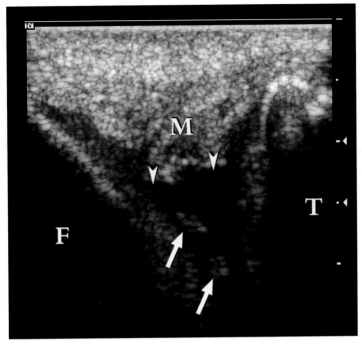

22a

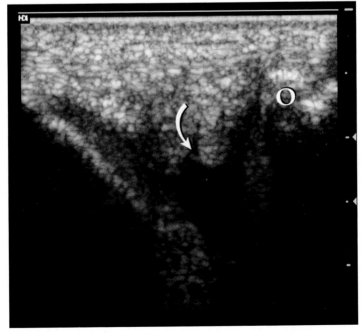

22b

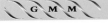

23: LS Coronal Oblique Postero-Medial Knee

A well defined almost anechoic area with an echogenic capsule (arrowheads) is demonstrated apparently extending from the periphery of the medial meniscus (M). The cystic structure has a broad base over the medial joint-line but proximally it appears to merge with the medial joint capsule (arrows). The medial meniscus itself appears normal.

Diagnosis:

Ganglion of the medial joint capsule (surgically proven).

Key point:

Although most cysts at the level of the media meniscus l are meniscal cysts, in this case the medial meniscus is clearly demonstrated and there is no evidence of a meniscal tear (these usually being of the horizontal cleavage type). Without such a tear then the cyst cannot be a true "meniscal cyst" and therefore in this case a "ganglion cyst" was the more likely diagnosis.

24: LS Coronal Oblique Antero-Lateral Knee

A hypoechoic fissure (arrowheads) within the meniscus (M) extending towards a hypoechoic area at its periphery (arrows) this latter area having a wall of variable echogenicity.

Diagnosis:

Horizontal cleavage tear lateral meniscus with secondary small meniscal cyst.

Key point:

The one-way-valve effect of the tears often results in stasis within the cyst and debris accumulaton this being reflected by the variations in echogenicity of such cysts.

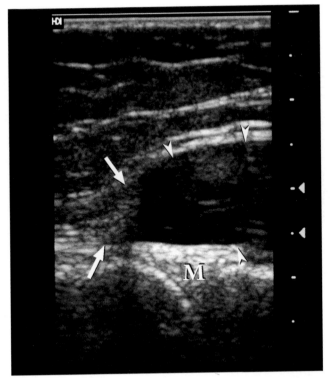

23

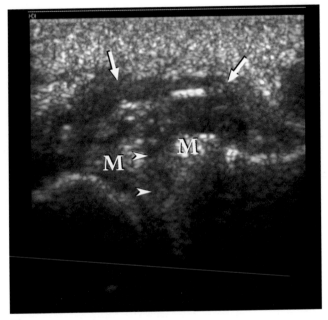

24

25: TS Postero-Medial Knee

There is a crescenteric fluid collection lying between the medial head of gastrocnemius (G) and the semimebranosus tendon (S) anterior to the posterior aspect of the medial femoral condyle (F). A septal band of synovium is present medially (arrow).

Diagnosis:

Simple popliteal (Baker's) cyst.

Key points:

1) A Baker's cyst by definition must extend out from the interspace between the medial head of gastrocnemius and semimembranosus. Although the bulk of the cyst may lie superficial or deep to the medial head of gastrocnemius or may extend almost entirely medial to semimembranosus it must be in continuity with this interspace at some point.

2) The synovial wall may demonstrate the features of synovitis seen elsewhere in the knee (see Fig 27a and 27b). Echogenic foci may be present within the cyst wall probably reflecting crystal deposition.

3) If there is stasis of the synovial fluid echogenic debris may not uncommonly be present and there may be calcific loose-bodies within the synovial fluid.

4) The volume of synovial fluid may increase if the patient is moved from the usual prone scanning position to a supine scanning position as synovial fluid passes from the knee joint into the dependent cyst. This communication, however, may only be unidirectional.

26: TS Postero-Medial Knee

A well defined anechoic structure (C) is seen lying superficial to the proximal metaphysis of tibia (T). This cyst is seen to be lying within rather than displacing the popliteus muscle (P) with a thin rim of muscle seen around the cyst especially anteriorly (arrowheads). Colour-doppler study did not demonstrate any abnormal vascularity within or surrounding this cyst. The cyst is separate from the medial head of gastrocnemius and there is no communication with the crescent surface of that structure.

Diagnosis:

Intramuscular ganglion of popliteus muscle.

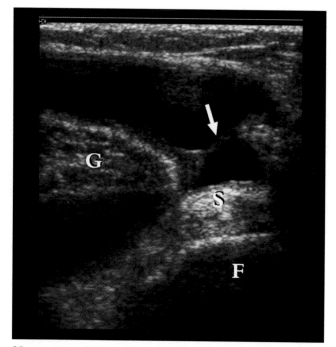

25

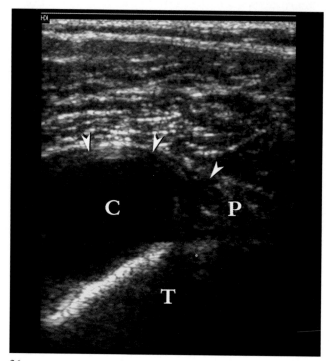

26

27a: LS Sagittal Midline Supra-Patella Pouch

Split-screen image demonstrating markedly thickened hypoechoic synovium (between arrowheads) lying between the quadriceps expansion (Q) and the supra-patella fat pad (P)/femur (F). An anechoic fissure is present within this thickened synovium representing a knee joint effusion (E) (left-hand image) which is effaced on increased compression (right-hand image).

27b: LS Sagittal Medial Supra-Patella Pouch

Split screen image in another patient. Again there is thickened/hypertrophic synovium but this time it has a fronded surface (arrowheads). The appearance of these fronds change as they float within the gently eddying synovial fluid, explaining the surface changes between right- and left-hand images (much better demonstrated in real-time).

Diagnosis:

Knee joint synovitis.

Key points:

1) Joint effusions are not static. If the supra-patella pouch is scanned during active knee flexion fluid may be compressed onto this area distending the pouch in mid-flexion while fluid may not be seen in this area during static extension or flexion. Similarly any fronds or septa may be seen to gently move akin to seaweed in a rock-pool.

2) Colour doppler imaging will often demonstrate prominent dilated vessels at the periphery or centrally within inflamed synovium.

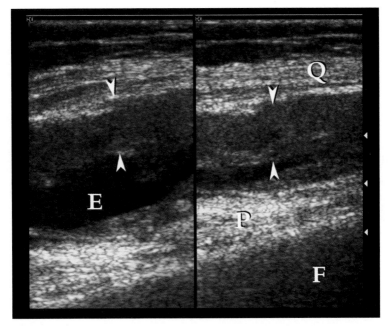

27a

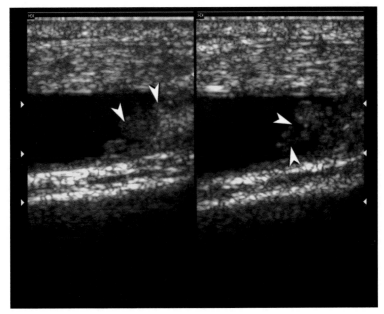

27b

28: LS Midline Proximal Calf

There is an area of anechoic fluid (H) dissecting between the more superficial gastrocnemius (G) and deeper soleus (S) muscles. There is no disruption of the normal muscle internal architecture.

Diagnosis:

The appearances could reflect either a dissecting haematoma or dissecting synovial fluid from a ruptured popliteal cyst.

Key points:

1) Careful examination of the popliteal fossa is indicated to look for proximal extension towards an abnormal semimembranosus/medial head of gastrocnemius bursa.

2) Lower limb sonovenographic study should be performed as secondary venous thrombus formation is not uncommon following either calf muscle haematoma or muscle tear or Baker's cyst rupture.

29: LS Postero-Medial Distal Thigh

The typical normal muscle architecture as seen on longitudinal section is generally evident, i.e. there is a "herring-bone" pattern of hypoechoic skeletal muscle bundles separated by longitudinally aligned echogenic connective tissue (epimysium). The scan plane is through the distal semimembranosus muscle. There is a small (<1cm) area of decreased echogenicity superficially (arrowheads) which does not contain echogenic epimysium and which slightly bulges the thick echogenic band of superficial fascia (arrows). Compression of this area showed it to be locally tender, i.e. reproduced characteristic pain.

Diagnosis:

Small peripheral tear of distal semimembranosus.

Key points:

1) The deeper muscle fibres run in a slightly different line to the superficial fibres, which is a common arrangement within a particular muscle.

2) The appearances of the muscle tear are non-specific in such cases and distinction from small soft-tissue tumours often lies more in the associated clinical history. Colour-flow doppler does not usually help as healing tears may or may not exhibit hyperaemia. Similarly tumours demonstrate variable new vessel formation.

3) In transverse section the epimysium is seen end-on and therefore appears as echogenic "dots" rather than "dashes" between the otherwise featureless hypoechoic muscle.

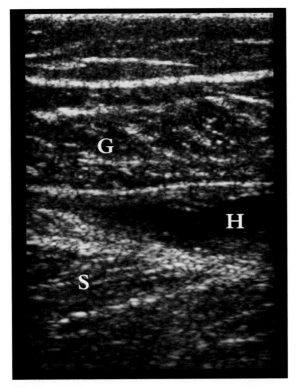

28

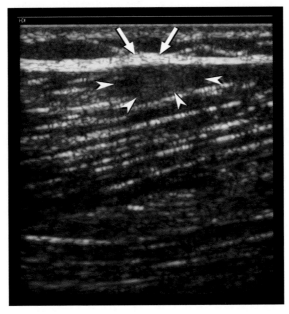

29

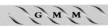

30: TS Oblique Anterior Axillary Wall

There is disruption of the costal head of pectoralis major (CO) with medial retraction of frayed muscle ends (arrow) and a resulting gap haematoma (H). The sternal head of pectoralis major (S) is relatively normal while the clavicular head (CL) demonstrates a heterogenous region more laterally (curved arrow).

Diagnosis:

Extensive partial rupture pectoralis major muscle.

Key point:

The percentage cross-sectional area of a muscle tear is important. A relatively small tear at this site may reflect a more extensive disruption of effective cross-sectional area than a much larger tear more medially.

31: LS Sagittal Anterior Aspect Middle Third Upper Arm

There is a markedly disorganised biceps brachialis muscle internal architecture proximally and a fluid collection (haematoma) more distally (H). Within the area of muscle disorganisation there are developing small foci of echogenic material (arrows) some of which exhibit acoustic shadowing (arrowheads).

Diagnosis:

Early myositis ossificans within a recent partial rupture biceps brachialis muscle.

Key point:

Myositis ossificans may be demonstrated on ultrasound as early as 7–10 days post injury, i.e. before CT and conventional radiography. Initially it appears as echogenic foci which later start to cast an acoustic shadow as aggregation progresses and calcific particle density increases. The ossification process is centripetal, i.e. it starts at the periphery and extends centrally (unlike tumoral calcinosis which is centrifugal). Mature ossification may appear as a solid mass (circumscripta form) or follow the line of muscle fibres.

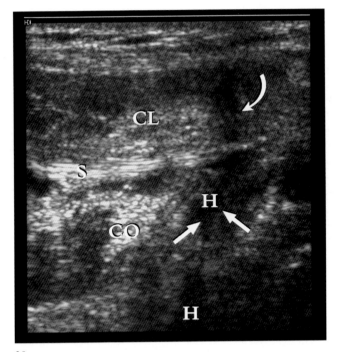

30

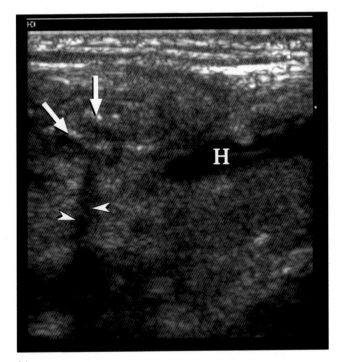

31

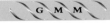

32: LS Sagittal Middle Finger at level of Proximal Interphalangeal Joint

The volar surfaces of 3rd proximal phalangeal head (H) and base of middle phalanx (B) are clearly identified as a landmark for changes in the overlying soft tissues. The flexor digitorum profundus tendon (F) is normal. (The flexor digitorum superficialis tendon is not seen in this section as it has undergone its normal split around the profunda tendon to insert into the base of middle phalanx para-sagitally.) Irregular pockets of fluid are present within the flexor tendon sheath (arrowheads) as well as a small intracapsular effusion within the proximal interphalangeal joint (curved arrow). The overlying volar soft tissues are thickened and oedematous with accentuation of the flexor skin crease.

Diagnosis:

Flexor tenosynovitis with small associated effusion (probably sympathetic).

Key point:

Although the tendon sheath fluid (and joint effusion) is anechoic, ultrasound is unable to distinguish accurately between simple fluid and thin pus therefore needle aspiration under ultrasound guidance should be considered depending on clinical circumstances. Alternately if a non-infected tenosynovitis is likely steroid injection may be more appropriate, this also being easily performed under ultrasound guidance.

33: Coronal LS Proximal Interphalangeal Joint (PIPJ) Middle Finger

There is a pit (curved arrow) in the bony surface of the base of middle phalanx (M). This pit is filled by almost anechoic soft-tissue. A hypoechoic triangle of tissue is present deep to the echogenic medial joint capsule (arrowheads), between the head of proximal phalanx (P) and the base of middle phalanx (M).

Diagnosis:

Rheumatoid type corner erosion and synovitis of PIPJ.

Key points:

1) The soft tissue within the marginal erosion is filled with rheumatoid pannus.

2) There is thickened, decreased echogenicity synovium generally.

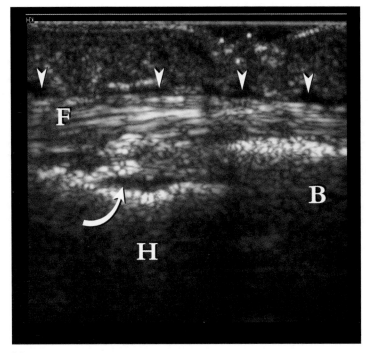

32

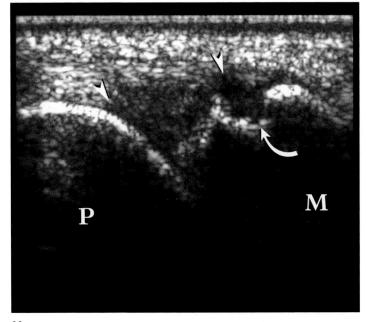

33

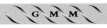

34: TS and LS Flexor Tendon Sheath Mid-Palm

The normal flexor tendons are more clearly demonstrated than normal due to the large volume of surrounding synovial fluid resulting in enhancement from its "water-bath" effect. In transverse section the separate superficial (flexor digitorum superficialis) and deep (flexor digitorum profundus) tendons produce a "figure-of-eight" appearance. In longitudinal section due to the scan plane adopted only the profunda tendon is seen.

Diagnosis:

Flexor tenosynovitis of mechanical origin mid-palmar region.

Key points:

1) There is remarkably little surrounding oedema, the synovial fluid is anechoic and synovial thickening is mild and regular. These features suggest sepsis to be of relatively low probability.

2) Increased transducer pressure did not elicit significant local tenderness. Ultrasound not only allows demonstration of abnormalities but also allows the opportunity to compress that region accurately to see if this reproduces or accentuates the patient's characteristic symptoms, i.e. ultrasound may be considered an extension of physical examination.

3) The distal end of the distended flexor tendon sheath has a "tear-drop" appearance due to limitation by a relatively fixed portion possibly at the site of fibrosis or vincula (nutrient vessel attachment).

35: LS and TS Radial Aspect Dorsum Wrist

Split-screen left-hand image shows a tortuous hypoechoic area (arrowheads) extending from a bulbous subcutaneous area (arrows) down to the hypoechoic joint capsule superficial to the radius (R)/scaphoid (S) joint. The right-hand image shows this serpiginous area (arrowheads) to be lateral and separate from radial artery (A).

Diagnosis:

Dorsal capsular ganglion.

Key point:

Ganglia have a tendency for production of complex meandering tracts with resultant difficulties in complete excision.

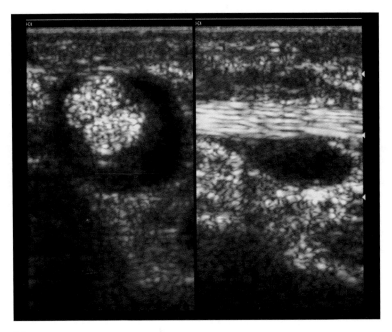

34

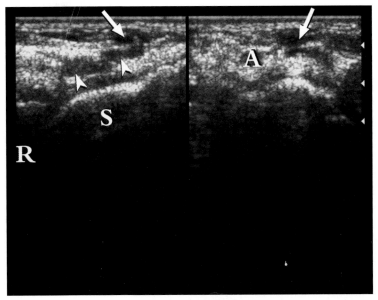

35

36a: LS Sagittal Mid-Line Volar Aspect of Wrist

The median nerve is seen as a well defined linear structure which is of normal echogenicity distally superficial to the volar surface of the lunate (L) with a fusiform thickening and decreased echogenicity (arrowheads) superficial to the distal radius (R).

36b: TS Volar Aspect Both Wrists

The elliptical normal right-hand median nerve (N) configuration becomes flattened and elongated in its transverse axis on the left hand. Normal flexor tendons (T) are seen deep to the median nerves bilaterally.

Diagnosis:

Carpal tunnel syndrome.

Key points:

1) The internal fibrillar pattern of nerves is more regular than that seen in tendons and a greater amount of hypoechoic tissue is seen between the neuronal bundles.

2) Sonographic features of carpal tunnel syndrome include :-

   i) Nerve swelling proximal to the compression point (36a).

   ii) Flattening of the nerve beneath compression point (36b).

   iii) Increased palmar bowing of the flexor retinaculum (arrows) (36b).

   iv) Decrease flexor tendon movement deep to the median nerve.

   v) Occasionally ganglia may be seen within the tunnel.

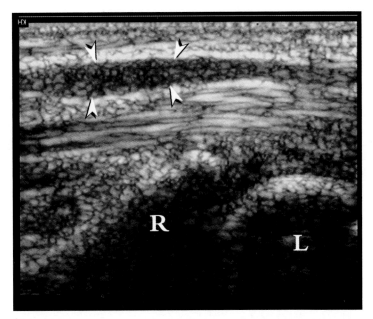

36a

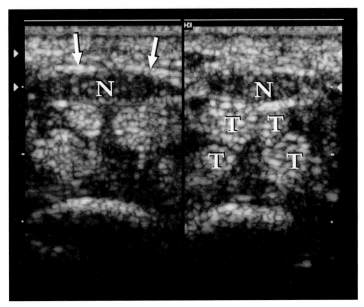

36b

37a: LS Sagittal Anterior Right Elbow

The medial nerve (arrowheads) just distal to the elbow joint is fusiformly thickened. In addition the internal linear fascicular pattern is more prominent due to increased interface separation. The nerve is crossed by a number of collateral vessels (arrow).

37b: LS Sagittal Anterior Right Elbow
(5mm lateral to the plane of median nerve)

There is an echogenic walled vessel (G) anterior to a normally walled artery (P) and separated by a dilated area (A) from a further normally walled vessel distally (D). Colour-flow doppler showed all of the above vessels to demonstrate arterial flow.

Diagnosis:

1) Post-traumatic neuroma of the median nerve.
2) False aneurism at the site of anastomosis of synthetic arterial graft to the distal brachial artery.
3) Collateral arterial circulation formation extending from native proximal brachial artery.

Key points:

1) The brachial artery required reconstruction following injury at time of median nerve decompression.
2) Synthetic arterial grafts usually have more echogenic walls than native vessels.

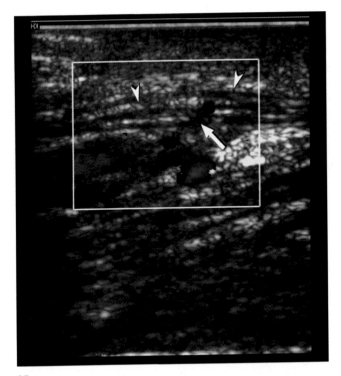

37a

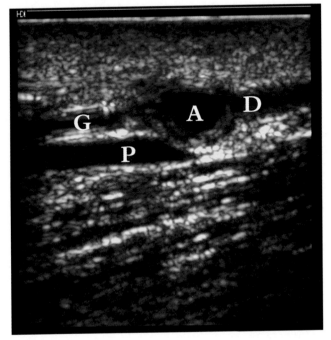

37b

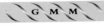

38: LS Coronal Oblique Antero-Medial Elbow

There are a series of well defined and separate tendons (here flexor carpi radialis [F]) of variable length to their musculo-tendinous junctions. The tendon origins are superficial to the medial epicondyle of humerus (M), medial border of trochlea (T) and medial articular process of proximal ulna (U). The echogenic medial elbow joint capsule (arrowheads) separates the tendons from bone surfaces.

Diagnosis:

Normal common flexor origin.

39: LS Coronal Oblique Antero-Lateral Elbow

The common tendon origin is difficult to separate into their individual tendon components, here the region of the extensor carpi radialis (E). It is also usually difficult to separate the normal tendon origins from the deeper lateral joint capsule, these lying superficial to the lateral epicondyle of humerus (L), lateral border of capitellum (C) and the radial head (R).

Diagnosis:

Normal common extensor origin.

Key point:

It is for the above anatomical regions that the specific tendon or capsular injury is more easily defined at the common flexor origin rather than at the common extensor origin.

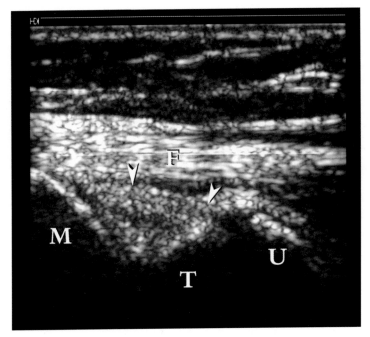

38

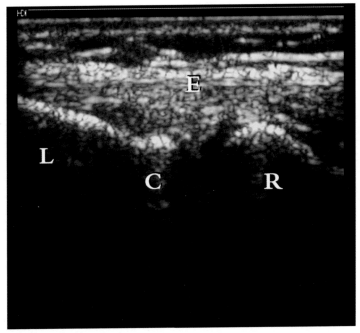

39

40: LS Coronal Oblique Antero-Lateral Elbow

There is a thickened, heterogenous anterolateral common extensor origin. The abnormal area represents the tendinous origin of the extensor carpi radialis longus and brevis tendons. These specific tendon origins are abnormal particularly its deep fibres (arrowheads). (The remaining common extensor origin appeared normal.) There is a small central tear developing (curved arrow).

Diagnosis:

"Tennis elbow".

Key point:

The specific site of tendinosis, i.e. antero-lateral common extensor origin, is typical of tennis elbow. Occasionally the lateral joint capsule may also be thickened.

41: LS Coronal Oblique Antero-Lateral Elbow

There is an irregular surface to the lateral epicondyle of humerus (arrowheads) with a small separate area of calcification superficially. The adjacent tendons of the common extensor origin are oedematous.

Diagnosis:

Lateral epicondylitis.

Key point:

Both of the above diagnoses are repetitive traction phenomena and these changes are often present in the same elbow.

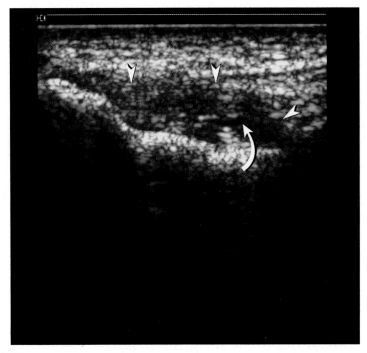

40

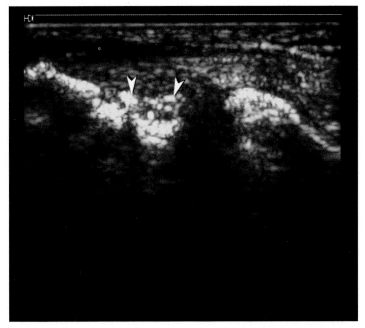

41

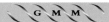

42: TS and LS Antero-Lateral Proximal Humerus
(at level of bicipital groove)

The images show fluid collection with a well defined synovial lined structure (arrowheads) with internal synovial septation, lying anterior to the biceps tendon (B) in both transverse (left) and longitudinal (right) planes. A thin layer of thickened synovium/fluid is present surrounding the long head of biceps tendon.

Diagnosis:

Subdeltoid bursitis.

Key points:

1) In the transverse axis in particular the transverse bicipital ligament (curved arrow) is seen to separate the subdeltoid bursa (arrowheads) from the biceps tendon sheath.

2) Subdeltoid bursitis is usually associated with rotator cuff disease and an isolated bursitis is rare.

3) An infective bursitis is usually secondary to needle inoculation or extension of a shoulder septic arthritis via a full-thickness rotator cuff tear.

43: LS Antero-Lateral Proximal Humerus

There is a mass of complex internal echogenicity with well defined superficial margin (arrowheads) displacing and thinning the overlying deltoid muscle (M). The underlying bony surface of proximal humerus is scalloped (arrows). Bone spicules extend into the mass and there is irregularity of the cortical surface more proximally (curved arrows).

(Colour-doppler study also demonstrated new-vessel formation both centrally within mass as well as at its periphery.)

Diagnosis:

Aggressive soft tissue neoplasm ? exact nature (in this case subperiosteal areast metastasis).

Key point:

Ultrasound will usually demonstrate whether a mass is present but with a few exceptions the appearances are non-specific and it may be difficult to even distinguish between benign and malignant tumours. Ultrasound does, however, allow excellent guidance of needle position for percutaneous biopsy.

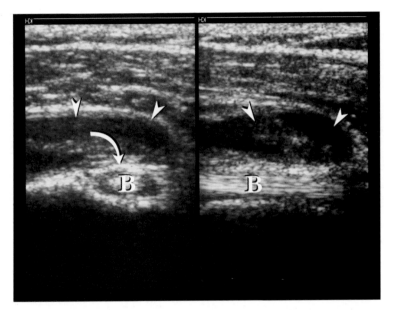

42

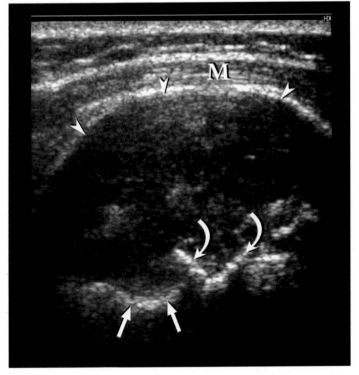

43

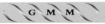

44a: Oblique Coronal Left Supraspinatus Tendon
(initial study)

A small hypoechoic fissure extends through the full thickness of the anterior portion of the supraspinatus tendon close to its periphery (curved arrow). The remaining tendon otherwise appears normal.

Diagnosis:

Small full thickness peripheral tear.

44b: Oblique Coronal Left Supraspinatus Tendon
(same patient 12 months later)

The previous fissure has become wider and the supraspinatus tendon (S) has moved medially towards the acromion (out of screen). A concavity is now present in the subdeltoid areolar soft-tissue overlying the apparent cuff defect (arrows).

Diagnosis:

Larger full thickness tear/peripheral detachment now with tendon retraction.

Key point:

The superficial surface of the supraspinatus tendon should be convex. A concave superficial surface infers a supraspinatus tear which is a useful secondary sign of tear when diagnosing tendon tears may be otherwise difficult, e.g. within tendinosis.

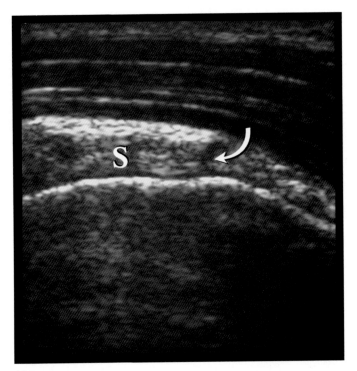

44a

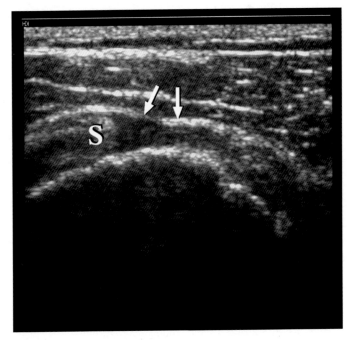

44b

45: Oblique Coronal Left Supraspinatus Tendon

There is pitting (arrow) of the superior surface of the proximal humerus/greater tuberosity (H) suggesting previous sub-acromial impingement. No demonstrable supraspinatus tendon is seen beneath the subdeltoid areolar connective tissue.

Diagnosis:

Massive rotator cuff tear with supraspinatus tendon retraction below the acromion process (A).

Key point:

The inexperienced observer often finds it surprisingly difficult to realise when there is a complete absence of the supraspinatus tendon, especially as the echogenic subdeltoid areolar connective tissue can look like a very thin supraspinatus tendon.

46: Oblique Coronal Right Supraspinatus Tendon (Anterior)

There is a markedly decreased/heterogenous echogenicity anterior supraspinatus tendon particularly laterally at the tendon periphery (arrowheads). A thin echogenic line is present superficial to the surface of the supero-lateral peripheral margin of the humeral head (arrow) – this later line represents the hyaline articular cartilage surface.

Diagnosis:

Supraspinatus tear within a generally degenerate tendon.

Key point:

The articular cartilage of the humeral head is not usually particularly well seen. The demonstration of an interface at this cartilage's superficial surface implies that there is fluid adjacent to that cartilage. In the absence of a joint effusion or if such an interface sign is only present over a small area of humeral head the demonstration of such an interface almost inevitably reflects an overlying cuff tear. Such an interface sign can be extremely useful in demonstrating a tear within an otherwise hypoechoic degenerate tendon. An interface is not seen more laterally, however, as the articular cartilage does not exist at site of osseo-tendinous junctions. This explains why in the current example such an interface sign does not exist at the tendon periphery even though it is likely that at least a partial tear has occurred in this region, considering the particularly marked tendon heterogeneity.

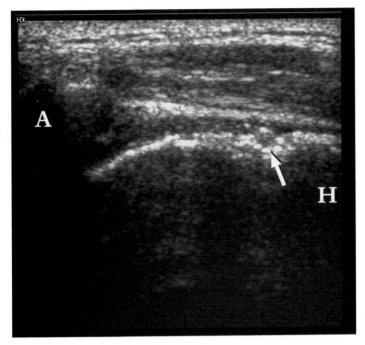

45

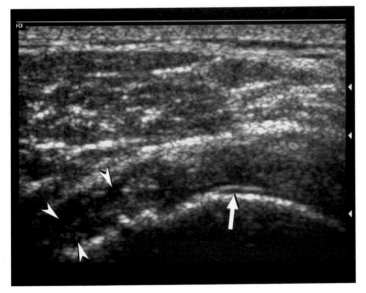

46

47a: Oblique Coronal Right Supraspinatus Tendon

The supraspinatus tendon (S) demonstrates decreased/heterogenous echogenicity particularly superficially and laterally. There is slight tendon thickening.

47b: Oblique Coronal Right Supraspinatus Tendon

(posterior to scan plane used in Fig 47a)

There is marked irregularity and pitting of the superior surface greater tuberosity of humerus (arrows). In addition there is a subtle horizontal cleavage tear developing (arrowheads) within the substance of the supraspinatus tendon.

Diagnosis:

Rotator cuff degeneration secondary to sub-acromial impingement.

Key points:

1) It may be difficult to distinguish between a partial and small, non-retracted full thickness tear within an otherwise degenerate tendon.

2) Dynamic study of shoulder abduction in sub-acromial impingement may also demonstrate:-

   i) Fluid extrusion from the sub-acromial bursa into the sub-deltoid bursa more laterally.

   ii) Bunching-up or pinching of the lateral third of supraspinatus tendon with consequent "blocking" of gleno-humeral movement at approximately 60 degrees of abduction (all further abduction being scapulo-thoracic movement rather than gleno-humeral).

   iii) A palpable "clunk" below, and felt through the transducer head.

(All of these features are best demonstrated with the dynamic study performed while abducting the shoulder from an initial position of internal rotation/adduction with the transducer in the oblique coronal plane (i.e. the same plane as for the above studies).

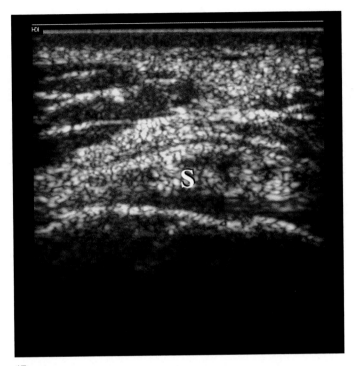

47a

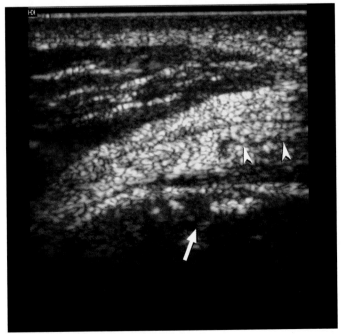

47b

48: TS Long Head of Biceps Tendon

The biceps tendon (B) demonstrates slightly decreased echogenicity centrally. The tendon has lost its normal rounded cross-section, i.e. there is tendon flattening suggesting "softening". The synovial sheath (arrowheads) is markedly thickened but with some internal echoes and is non-compressible with increased transducer pressure consistent with synovitis rather than simple fluid distension.

Diagnosis:

Biceps tenosynovitis.

Key points:

1)˙ A long head of biceps tendon often becomes flattened "normally" in its intra-articular portion above the level of the bicipital groove although such flattening may occur secondary to tendon degeneration. Flattening distal to the bicipital groove as seen here is usually abnormal.

2) Complex synovial fluid may contain internal echoes, however, fluid is "ballottable" with compression whereas synovial thickening is relatively non-compressible.

3) 90–95% of patients with a rotator cuff tear also have at least a small effusion within the biceps tendon sheath.

49: LS and TS Left Long Head of Biceps Tendon (at inferior end of bicipital groove)

There is a relatively well-defined focus of decreased echogenicity (arrows) extending along the longitudinal axis of an otherwise normal biceps tendon. A thickened synovial tendon sheath is present but without fluid within this sheath.

Diagnosis:

Longitudinal shear tear and mild associated tenosynovitis.

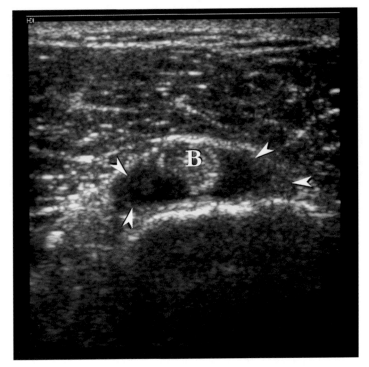

48

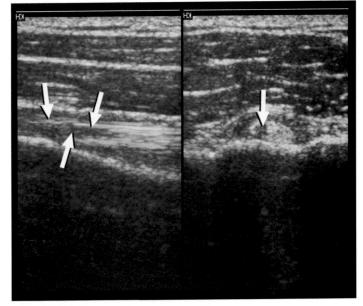

49

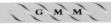

50: LS Bicipital Groove

There is an echogenic focus (arrowheads) lying within the biceps tendon sheath anterior/superficial to the long head of biceps tendon with posterior acoustic shadowing. The tendon itself images normally.

Diagnosis:

Calcific tenosynovitis.

Key point:

This is a common site for calcium hydroxyapetite deposition. It is the author's experience that such calcification is much more common than a true calcific tendonitis (unless there has been previous steroid injection).

51: TS Mid Bicipital Groove

The long head of biceps brachialis tendon (B) lies medial to the bicipital groove (arrows). The groove is filled by fluid and a small amount of echogenic debris. The echogenic transverse bicipital ligament appears intact at least laterally (arrowheads) but could possibly be partially deficient medially.

Diagnosis:

Medial dislocation of long head of biceps tendon.

Key points:

1) A dynamic study in internal/external rotation should routinely be performed of the bicipital groove and biceps tendon. A medially displaced tendon in external rotation may relocate in neutral or internal rotation.

2) Biceps tendons dislocate medially. Usually the transverse bicipital ligament is intact and the biceps migrates medially beneath the subscapularis which becomes detached from its insertion on the lesser tuberosity of humerus. More rarely the transverse ligament ruptures and the biceps tendon displaces antero-medially, superficial to the subscapularis tendon.

3) If a significant amount of synovial debris remains in the groove following long head of biceps tendon dislocation (or rupture) a "pseudo-biceps tendon" appearance can occur.

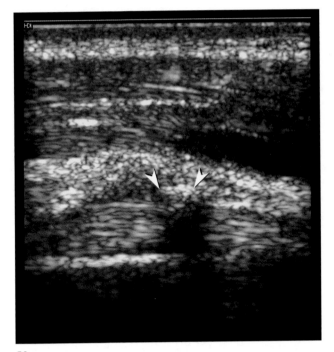

50

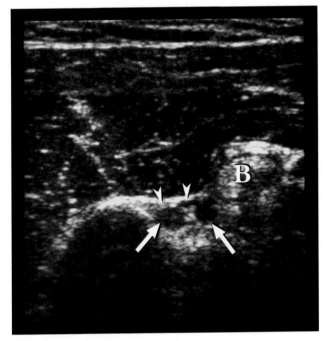

51

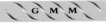

REFERENCES

1. Aisen A M, McCune W J, MacGuire A, Carson P L, Silver T M, Jafri S Z, Martel W. Sonographic Evaluation of the Cartilage of the Knee. *Radiology* 153:781-784,1984.

2. Berman L, Fink A M, Wilson D, McNally E. Technical Note: Identifying and Aspirating Hip Effusions. *The British Journal of Radiology* 68:306-310, 1995.

3. Bertolotto M, Perrone R, Martinoli C, Rollandi G A, Patetta R, Derchi L E. High Resolution Ultrasound Anatomy of Normal Achilles Tendon. *The British Journal of Radiology* 68:986-991, 1995.

4. Bianchi S, Abdelwahab I F, Maxxola C G, Ricci G, Damiani S. Sonographic Examination of Muscle Herniation. *J Ultrasound Med* 14:357-360, 1995.

5. Bianchi S, Zwass A, Abdelwahab I F, Mazzola C G, Olivier M, Rettagliata F. Sonographic Evaluation of Intramuscular Ganglia. *Clinical Radiology* 50:235-236, 1995.

6. Bianchi S, Zwass A, Abdelwahab I F, Ricci G, Rettagliata F, Olivieri M. Sonographic Evaluation of Lipohemarthrosis: Clinical and In Vitro Study. *J Ultrasound Med* 14:279-282, 1995.

7. Bradley M, Bhamra M S, Robson M J. Ultrasound Guided Aspiration of Symptomatic Supraspinatus Calcific Deposits. *The British Journal of Radiology* 68:716-719, 1995.

8. Brophy D P, Cunnane G, Fitzgerald O, Gibney R G. Technical Report: Ultrasound Guidance for Injection of Soft Tissue Lesions Around the Heel in Chronic Inflammatory Arthritis. *Clinical Radiology* 50:120-122, 1995.

9. Buchberger W, Judmaier W, Birbamer G, Lener M, Schmidauer C. Carpal Tunnel Syndrome: Diagnosis with High-Resolution Sonography. *Am J Roentgen* 159:793-798, October 1992.

10. Chan T W, Dalinka M K, Kneeland J B, Chevrot A. Biceps Tendon Dislocation: Evaluation with MR Imaging. *Radiology* 179:649-652, 1991.

11. Crass J R, Craig E V, Feinberg S B. Ultrasonography of Rotator Cuff Tears: A Review of 500 Diagnostic Studies. *J Clin Ultrasound* 16:313-327, June 1988.

12. De Flaviis L, Nessi R, Leonardi M, Ulivi M. Dynamic Ultrasonography of Capsulo-Ligamentous Knee Joint Traumas. *J Clin Ultrasound* 16:487-492, September 1988.

13. Farin P U, Jaroma H, Harju A, Soimakallio S. Shoulder Impingement Syndrome: Sonographic Evaluation. *Radiology* 176:845-849, 1990.

14. Farin P U, Jaroma H. Sonographic Findings of Rotator Cuff Calcifications. *J Ultrasound Med* 14:7-14, 1995.

15. Fornage B D, Schernberg F L, Rifkin M D. Ultrasound Examination of the Hand. *Radiology* 1985; 155:785-788.

16. Howden M D. Foreign Bodies Within Finger Tendon Sheaths Demonstrated by Ultrasound: Two Cases. *Clinical Radiology* 49:419-420 (1994).

17. Jeffrey R B, Laing F C, Schechter W P, Markison R E, Barton R M. Acute Suppurative Tenosynovitis of the Hand: Diagnosis with US. *Radiology* 162:741-742, 1987.

18. Kainberger F M, Engel A, Barton P, Huebsch P, Neuhold A, Salomonowitz E. Injury of the Achilles Tendon: Diagnosis with Sonography. *Am J Roentgen* 155:1031-1036, November 1990.

19. Kaplan P A, Matamoros A, Anderson J C. Sonography of the Musculoskeletal System. *Am J Roentgen* 155:237-245, August 1990.

20. Katx T, Landman J, Dulitzky F, Bar-Ziv J. Fracture of the Clavicle in the Newborn: An Ultrasound Diagnosis. *J Ultrasound Med* 7:21-23, 1988.

21. Koski J M, Anttila P J, Isomäki H A. Ultrasonography of the Adult Hip Joint. *Scand J Rheumatology* 18:113-117, 1989.

22. Larcos G, Antico V F, Cormick W, Gruenewald S M, Farlow D C. How Useful is Ultrasonography in Suspected Acute Osteomyelitis? *J Ultrasound Med* 13:707-709, 1994.

23. Markowitz R I, Davidson R S, Harty M P, Bellah R D, Hubbard A M, Rosenberg H K. Sonography of the Elbow in Infants and Children. *Am J Roentgen* 159:829-833, October 1992.

24. Martinoli C, Derchi L E, Pastorino C, Bertolotto M, Silvestri E. Analysis of Echotexture of Tendons with US. *Radiology* 186:839-843, 1993.

25. McDonnell C H, Jeffrey R B, Björkengren A G, Li K C P. Intraarticular Sonography for Imaging the Knee Menisci: Evaluation in Cadaveric Specimens. *Am J Roentgen* 159:573-574, September 1992.

26. Middleton W D, Edelstein G, Reinus W R, Melson G L, Totty W G, Murphy W A. Sonographic Detection of Rotator Cuff Tears. *Am J Roentgen* 144:349-353, February 1985.

27. Morin C, Harcke H T, MacEwen. The Infant Hip: Real-Time UK Assessment of Acetabular Development. *Radiology* 157:673-677, 1985.

28. Nath A K, Arunchala U. Use of Ultrasound in Osteomyelitis. *The British Journal of Radiology* 65:649-652, 1992.

29. Odler J, Terrier B, von Schulthess G K, Fuchs W A. MRI and Sonography of the Shoulder. *Clinical Radiology* 43:323-327, 1991.

30. Olive R J, Marsh H E. Ultrasonography of Rotator Cuff Tears. *Clinical Orthopaedics and Related Research* 282: 110-113, 1992.

31. Özbek S S, Arkun R, Killi R, Memis A, Dagdeviren A, Sevinç E. Image-Directed Color Doppler Ultrasonography in the Evaluation of Superficial Solid Tumors. *J Clin Ultrasound* 23:233-238, May 1995.

32. Pai V R, van Holsbeeck M. Synovial Osteochondromatosis of the Hip: Role of Sonography. *J Clin Ultrasound* 23:199-203, March/April 1995.

33. Patten R M, Mack L A, Wang K Y, Lingel J. Nondisplaced Fractures of the Greater Tuberosity of the Humerus: Sonographic Detection. *Radiology* 182:201-204, 1992.

34. Rubaltelli L, Fiocco U, Cozzi L, Baldovin M, Rigon C, Bortoletto P, Tregnaghi A, Melanotte P L, di Maggio C, Todesco S. Prospective Sonographic and Arthroscopic Evaluation of Proliferative Knee Joint Synovitis. *J Ultrasound Med* 13:855-862, 1994.

35. Rupp S, Tempelhof S, Fritsch E. Ultrasound of the Achilles Tendon After Surgical Repair: Morphology and Function. *The British Journal of Radiology* 68: 454-458, 1995.

36. Selby B, Richardson M L, Nelson B D, Graney D O, Mack L A. Sonography in the Detection of Meniscal Injuries of the Knee: Evaluation in Cadavers. *Am J Roentgen* 149:549-553, September 1987

37. Selby B, Richardson M L, Montana M A, Teitz C C, Larson R V, Mack L A. High Resolution Sonography of the Menisci of the Knee. *High Resolution Sonography* 4; 332-335.

38. Shiels W E, Babcock D S, Wilson J L, Burch R A. Localisation and Guided Removal of Soft-Tissue Foreign Bodies with Sonography. *Am J Roentgen* 155:1277-1281, December 1990.

39. Takebayashi S, Takasawa H, Banzai Y, Miki H, Sasaki R, Itoh Y, Matsubara S. Sonographic Findings in Muscle Strain Injury: Clinical and MR Imaging Correlation. *J Ultrasound Med* 14:899-905, 1995.

INDEX